Lamine Ghanem Lakhal

Acute renal failure in intensive care

Lamine Ghanem Lakhal

Acute renal failure in intensive care

ScienciaScripts

Imprint
Any brand names and product names mentioned in this book are subject to trademark, brand or patent protection and are trademarks or registered trademarks of their respective holders. The use of brand names, product names, common names, trade names, product descriptions etc. even without a particular marking in this work is in no way to be construed to mean that such names may be regarded as unrestricted in respect of trademark and brand protection legislation and could thus be used by anyone.

Cover image: www.ingimage.com

This book is a translation from the original published under ISBN 978-3-8416-7735-8.

Publisher:
Sciencia Scripts
is a trademark of
Dodo Books Indian Ocean Ltd. and OmniScriptum S.R.L publishing group

120 High Road, East Finchley, London, N2 9ED, United Kingdom
Str. Armeneasca 28/1, office 1, Chisinau MD-2012, Republic of Moldova, Europe
Managing Directors: Ieva Konstantinova, Victoria Ursu
info@omniscriptum.com

Printed at: see last page
ISBN: 978-620-8-39807-1

ACUTE RENAL FAILURE IN INTENSIVE CARE

LAMINE GHANEM LAKHAL

Table of contents

1. INTRODUCTION :

Acute renal failure in the intensive care unit is an independent factor in mortality (1,2). The prevalence of acute renal failure in hemodynamically unstable ICU patients can be as high as 50% (2), using the classic criteria for defining acute renal failure (3,4). The reduction in glomerular filtration rate is expressed biologically by an accumulation of nitrogenous waste products (creatinine) and clinically by a reduction in diuresis.

The definition of renal dysfunction is based on the 2012 KDIGO criteria, which combine a clinical parameter represented by diuresis rate, and a biological parameter that assesses the variation in creatinine levels.

The use of renal perfusion as a method of assessing renal function is not recommended. Doppler measurement of the renal resistance index is mainly used to select, triage and prevent renal damage.

The classic etiological division of renal failure into pre-renal, renal and post-renal damage is valid in the ICU.

The severity of acute renal failure can be assessed using the same criteria that define acute renal injury. The "weight" parameter is not taken into account by the KDIGO criteria, the definition of AKI and the assessment of the severity of renal dysfunction in the paediatric population is made by the modified RIFLES criteria (p RIFLE).

Preventing AKI involves identifying subjects at risk, and optimizing systemic and locoregional hemodynamic conditions. The use of products with nephrotoxic potential must be carefully balanced in terms of benefit and risk.

Peri-operative renal failure is defined in the same way, with predominantly pre-renal and renal involvement. Post-renal involvement is not exceptional, and should be systematically ruled out in the presence of post-operative anuria, by simple ultrasound examination.

Treatment is symptomatic, pending regression of renal damage. Extra-renal purification is indicated in situations of overload, hyperkalemia and acidosis due to impaired renal acidifying capacity. Other indications should be discussed on a case-by-case basis.

The use of loop diuretics is not systematic, but should be considered in situations of hypervolemia and overload, and on a temporary basis.

The use of low-dose (renal dose) dopamine to vasodilate splanchnic territories and the renal afferent artery is not recommended.

If glomerular filtration rate (GFR) is to be estimated, the estimated formulas (Cockroft-Gault, MDRD, CKD-EPI) should not be used in intensive care or postoperative patients. The formula for calculating creatinine clearance (UV/P creatinine) should probably be used.

2. DEFINITIONS :

Current definitions use the KDIGO criteria, which, in addition to defining AKI, enable severity to be assessed using clinical-biological criteria (altered diuresis output and increased creatinine levels). It is therefore preferable to use a specific terminology that corresponds to the different stages of renal suffering, from aggression to damage and dysfunction (Figure 1) (5).

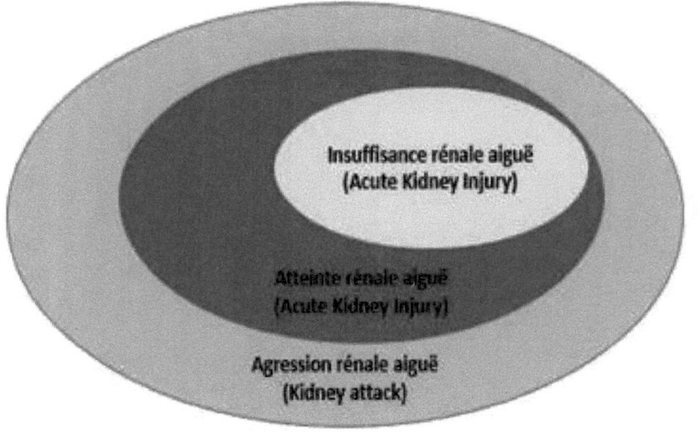

(5)

Figure 2: Acute renal failure: from aggression to dysfunction.

The limitations of creatinine in assessing filtration rate have been highlighted, making it an imperfect marker (dependent on muscle mass, late accumulation in relation to altered glomerular filtration rate (Figure 2) (5). However, the almost ubiquitous availability of plasma creatinine measurement, its low cost and familiarity with its use, make it the most cost-effective renal biomarker for defining acute renal failure (5).

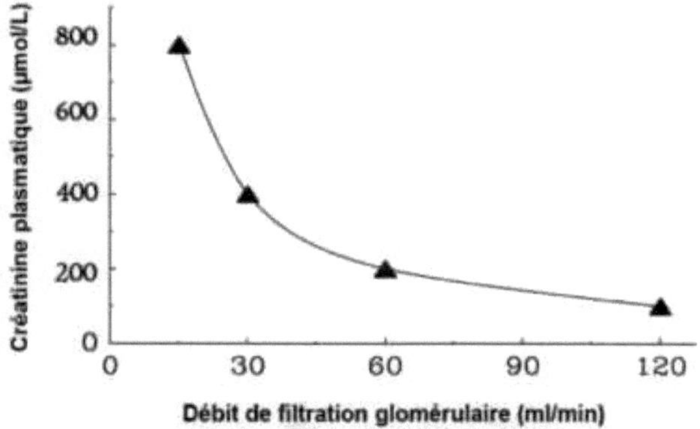

Figure 2: Relationship between glomerular filtration rate and creatinine levels

Urea levels depend not only on renal function, but also on many other parameters, making its measurement a poor biomarker of glomerular filtration (6). These parameters are represented by :

- Protein intake.
- Protein catabolism in the body.
- The person's state of hydration.
- Gastrointestinal bleeding.

There are also so-called physiological variations:

- Pregnancy reduces its concentration by 30-60%.
- Age: concentration falls in infants (-30%) and rises in adults over 55 (+20%).
- Gender: due to the difference in muscle mass, urea is higher in men than in women (5%).
- Prolonged effort can increase concentration by 20%.
- Prolonged fasting (significantly reduces urea concentration).

In the KDIGO criteria, at least one of the following three criteria must be present:

- Plasma creatinine increased by 26.5 mmol/L in 48 h.
- An increase in plasma creatinine of 1.5 times the baseline value within the last 7 days.
- Diuresis < 0.5 ml/kg/h for 6 h.

The KDIGO classification represents an optimized synthesis of two pre-existing combined classifications (RIFLE and AKIN), developed by international expert groups of nephrologists and resuscitators to characterize the severity of acute renal failure (84).

In children, the diagnosis of acute renal failure should probably be made using the pediatric-modified RIFLE classification (pRIFLE)(table 8).

There are other markers used much more to detect the mechanism of renal tissue aggression and not for the diagnosis of renal failure due to cost and lack of clinical studies, the best known of which are (7):

- Cystatin C.
- Kidney Injury molecule-1 (KIM-1).
- Neutrophil gelatinase associated lipocalin (NGAL).
- Interleukin-18 (IL-18).
- β2-microglobulin.

The study of renal perfusion by parenchymal pulsed Doppler, or by semi-quantitative assessment using color Doppler, or by renal contrast ultrasonography, appears to be a promising method for the early diagnosis of renal damage.

Advances in the use of non-invasive techniques (ultrasound) to diagnose and monitor various pathologies in emergency and intensive care settings have made it possible to study renal perfusion using the Doppler method, as part of the assessment of renal function.

The study of renal perfusion by renal parenchymal Doppler probably enables early detection of patients at risk of developing acute renal failure, so that so-called preventive strategies can be planned. (8)

Several methods of assessing renal perfusion can be used in renal ultrasound. They are represented by :

- The semi-quantitative color Doppler renal perfusion assessment scale.
- Contrast-enhanced ultrasound (CEUS).
- Renal vascular resistance index (RRI).

Semi-quantitative assessment using color Doppler allows us to determine a scale for evaluating renal perfusion, ranging from 0 (no identifiable vessels) to 3 (visible vessels up to the arterial arteries).

Ultrasound coupled with the injection of contrast-enhanced ultrasound (CEUS) enables the measurement of two indices: mean transit time and relative blood volume. A relationship between these two indices reflects visceral perfusion.

Human data highlight the heterogeneity of the results obtained and the lack of correlation between CEUS-derived indices and renal macro- or microcirculatory data (9).

The study of renal perfusion by pulsed Doppler allows the measurement of two indices:

- Renal resistance index (RRI) deduced from systolic and diastolic velocities

$$\text{Index de résistance rénal} = \frac{\text{Vitesse systolique} - \text{Vitesse diastolique}}{\text{Vitesse systolique}}$$

- The pulsatility index (PI), calculated from systolic, diastolic and mean velocities.

$$\text{Index de pulsatilité} = \frac{\text{Vitesse systolique} - \text{Vitesse diastolique}}{\text{Vitesse moyenne}}$$

The profile of the renal circulation is a non-resistive profile, and the use of the renal resistance index is the most appropriate, since the pulsatility index is used for circulations with a resistive profile (e.g. vessels of both upper and lower limbs).

The renal resistance index has been used as a diagnostic tool and prognostic indicator of acute renal failure in several studies. We find it as :

- Diagnosis of early renal graft rejection (10).
- Method for assessing the impact of ureteral obstruction on renal function (11).
- Technique for assessing the risk of postoperative renal failure (12).
- A prognostic indicator in acute renal failure (persistence or reversibility of AKI) (13).

Table 1 summarizes the various clinical situations described in the literature where a pathological renal resistance index may be observed (14).

Table 1: Renal resistance index and possible pathologies described in the literature :

Pathology	Renal resistance index	Suggested clinical value (14)
Nephropathies	>0,75	Indicator of tubulointerstitial nephropathy (15)
AKI (acute kidney injury)	>0,75	Differentiating between functional and organic damage (16)
Chronic renal failure	>0,80	Indicator of irreversible damage
Chronic renal failure	>0,70	Independent factor in worsening renal damage (17, 18)
Urinary obstruction	>0,70	Complete obstruction of urinary tract (10, 19)
Urinary obstruction	Delta IRR>0.08-0.10	
Kidney transplantation	>0,80	Poor prognostic factor for kidney transplantation (9)
Type 1 diabetes	>0,64 children < 15 years	Risk of diabetic nephropathy(20)
Type 2 diabetes	>0,70	Indicator of advanced glomerular damage and/or arteriosclerosis(21)
Type 2 diabetes	>0,73	Progressive diabetic nephropathy(22)
Renal artery stenosis	>0,80	Poor efficacy of percutaneous revascularization (13)
Cirrhosis of the liver	>0,78	Risk of hepatorenal syndrome (23)

The classic etiological classification into pre-renal, parenchymal and post-renal renal failure remains relevant in clinical practice. In intensive care, the etiologies of acute renal failure can be classified as follows (5):

- Acute functional renal failure (30-60%) due to reduced renal perfusion pressure or renal blood flow.
- Acute organic renal failure, where acute tubular necrosis predominates (80% of parenchymal causes).
- Acute obstructive renal failure is rarer in the intensive care setting (1-10%), but should be suspected and eliminated systematically by ultrasound.

3. FUNCTIONAL ACUTE RENAL FAILURE

Acute functional renal failure is secondary to a reduction in renal blood flow, which leads to renal parenchymal hypoperfusion, causing acute renal injury (25). This is a form of renal failure to be suspected in the clinical context (shock, dehydration, etc.), and the diagnosis of certainty is retrospective (return to previous renal function after re-establishment of normal renal perfusion). Functional acute renal failure can be caused by a number of etiologies:

3.1 True hypovolemia :

It corresponds to a real loss of intravascular fluid content (normal = 75 ml/kg), as in hemorrhage and dehydration.

3.2 Relative hypovolemia :

In certain clinical situations, there may be a mismatch between vascular content and container, with vasoplegia phenomena (peripheral vasodilatation) observed in septic states, anaphylactic reactions, or certain cardiotropic drug intoxications.

3.3 Myocardial dysfunction:

Alterations in myocardial pump performance, whether direct (ischemic heart disease, myocarditis) or indirect (tamponade), can lead to low peripheral flow and functional renal impairment.

3.4 Pre-glomerular vasoconstriction:

Preglomerular vasoconstriction can be induced by several factors:

3.4.1 ***Non-steroidal anti-inflammatory drugs (NSAIDs):***

Intra-glomerular hydrostatic pressure and glomerular filtration rate are dependent on permanent vasodilation of the glomerular afferent arteriole. This permanent dilation is due to the local production of vasodilatory prostacyclins, favored by situations of chronic renal aggression (hypovolemia, prolonged low flow, cirrhosis, etc.). Non-steroidal anti-inflammatory drugs inhibit cyclooxygenase (COX 1, COX2), and reduce prostaglandin synthesis, which limits vasodilation of the renal afferent arteriole and favors the tendency to vasoconstriction.

3.4.2 ***Use of vasoactive amines :***

The use of high doses of alpha adrenergic drugs promotes ischemic renal aggression (intense vasoconstriction in the renal perfusion territory).

3.4.3 ***Other factors influencing intra-renal Phdmodynamics :***

The use of certain drugs, such as cyclosporine, and hepatorenal syndrome, which induces the liver to produce vasodilatory mediators, are factors favoring renal hypoperfusion.

3.5 Post-glomerular vasodilation:

The use of ACE inhibitors and angiotensin II antagonists (ARBs) is the main cause of postglomerular vasodilation. Intra-glomerular pressure and glomerular filtration rate are dependent on permanent vasoconstriction of the glomerulus' efferent arteriole by a local action of angiotensin II. This action is favored by situations of RAAS (renin-angiotensin-aldosterone system) activation, such as hypovolemia, bilateral renal artery stenosis and aortic coarctation...

ACE inhibitors and sartans reduce the production or action of angiotensin II on its receptors, thus promoting vasodilation of the efferent arteriole and a secondary decrease in glomerular chamber pressure, which alters glomerular filtration rate.

4. ACUTE RENAL FAILURE

Type of description: acute tubular necrosis (ATN).

Acute tubular necrosis is responsible for 80% of acute parenchymal renal failure. In intensive care, several situations can lead to renal failure due to tubular necrosis:

- Prolonged renal ischemia.
- Inflammatory reactions and sepsis.
- Use of iodinated contrast media
- The use of certain antibiotics (aminoglycosides).
- Certain intoxications with nephrotoxic products (ethylene glycol, etc.).
- Rhabdomyolysis.

Three mechanisms dominate tubular damage:

- Ischemia.
- Direct cellular toxicity.
- Tubular obstruction.

The clinical context of acute renal failure is often suggestive. Diuresis is preserved in 40% of cases. Oligo-anuria is observed in 60% of cases, with a diuresis of less than 400 ml/24h, or even anuria (diuresis of less than 100 ml/24h). Acute tubular necrosis has many etiologies:

4.1 Tubular ischemia:

Tubular ischemia can occur in certain situations of prolonged hemodynamic stress and significant fluid loss:

- Dehydration.
- States of shock.
- Major surgery (abdominal aortic aneurysm, extracorporeal circulation).

4.2 Toxicity to tubular cells:

Tubular cell toxicity can be seen in several situations:

- Use of iodinated contrast media.
- The use of certain anti-infective agents (aminoglycosides, vancomycin, amphotericin B.).
- In certain types of intoxication (ecstasy, etc.).

Hemolysis and rhabdomyolysis are frequent etiologies of acute tubular necrosis in the emergency and intensive care setting:

4.2.1 Acute hemolysis:

Because of its size (34-69 kda), hemoglobin released during acute intravascular hemolysis is poorly filtered by glomeruli, but has a toxic effect on tubular cells.

4.2.2 Rhabdomyolysis:

When released into the bloodstream, myoglobin is freely filtered by the glomerulus due to its low molecular weight, and is endocytosed by tubular cells, where it exerts a direct toxicity. Myoglobin can induce renal hypoperfusion by local vasoconstriction, and can form tubular cylinders with an obstructive effect.

4.2.3 Aminoglycosides :

Aminoglycosides induce distal tubular dysfunction with impaired urine concentration. They are completely and freely filtered by the glomeruli. Some of these aminoglycosides are absorbed by the tubular cells, and due to the rapid saturation of this absorption, they accumulate in the lysosomes of the tubular cells and induce acute toxicity. Aminoglycoside nephrotoxicity is predictable, avoidable and, above all, reversible, compared to ototoxicity (if prescribed correctly).

4.2.4 Iodinated contrast medium :

Iodine-induced acute tubular necrosis could be explained by two mechanisms (Figure 3):

- Intense medullary vasoconstriction reduces tubular perfusion.
- Direct iodine toxicity on tubular epithelial cells.

Plasma creatinine rises immediately after injection, peaks after 48 hours and decreases from day 4ème onwards. Renal failure is often diuresis preserved, rarely oligo-auric. To reduce the risk of iodine toxicity, it is first necessary to assess the usefulness of the radiological examination and the injection of the iodine product, and to evaluate subjects at risk by stopping medications that may aggravate renal damage. Some suggest rehydration regimens using crystalloid solutions (3 ml/kg one hour before and 12 ml/kg over the six hours following the examination). The benefits of iodine dialysis have been demonstrated by some, but not by others.

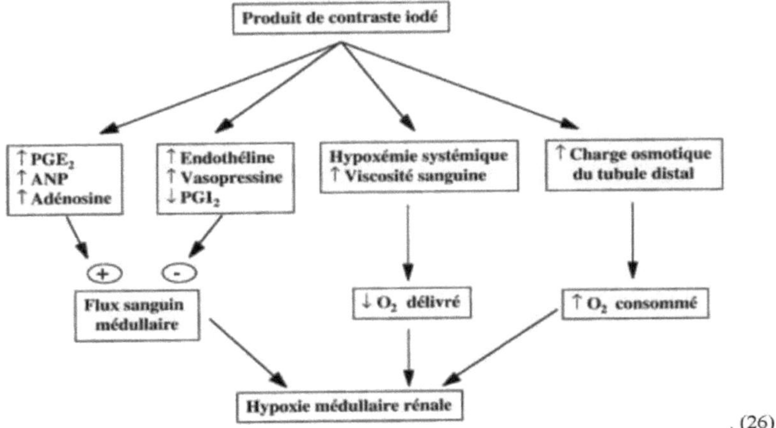

. (26)

Figure 3: Toxicity of iodinated contrast media.

4.2.5 The phenomena of tubular obstructions:

Certain drugs used in intensive care can cause tubular obstruction (Acyclovir, methotrexate). Ethylene glycol intoxication is another etiology of obstruction.

5. ACUTE OBSTRUCTIVE RENAL FAILURE

All cases of acute renal failure require renal ultrasound to rule out obstructive causes. The presence of pyelo-calicel dilatation is probably a sign of obstructive renal failure (Figure 4). The absence of urinary tract dilatation makes obstructive acute renal failure unlikely, without ruling it out completely (sensitivity 85%). False negatives may be due to recent obstruction, retroperitoneal fibrosis or severe dehydration. In intensive care and emergency patients, always look for iatrogenic obstructions on urinary catheters.

Functional obstructions, which are often reversible, are observed after morphine administration and central medullary anesthesia.

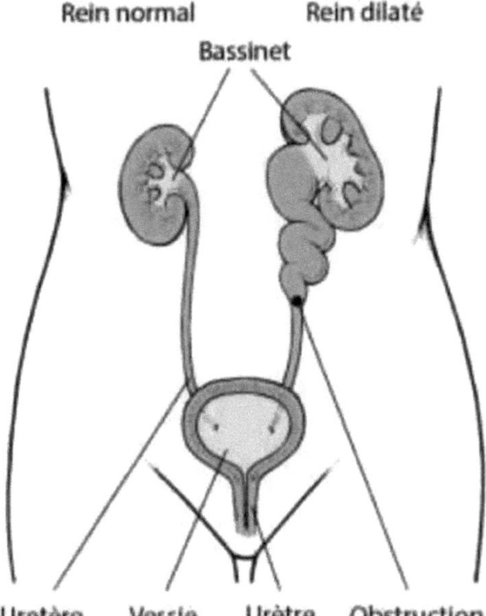

Figure 4: Dilatation of pyelo-calicelar cavities in organic obstructions

The pathophysiology of intratubular obstructions differs from that of acute excretory tract obstructions. In tubular obstructions, the tubules are dilated and the pressure regime in the excretory tract is normal; in the second situation, the stresses exerted on the walls are considerable, leading to deformation of the pyelocecal cavities, while intra-tubular pressures are nevertheless high, resulting in alteration of the glomerular ultrafiltrate (27).

6. ASSESSING THE SEVERITY OF ACUTE RENAL FAILURE

The severity of acute renal failure is always assessed using the KDIGO criteria. This classification (Table 2) represents a synthesis of the two classic pre-existing combined classifications (RIFLE and AKIN), developed by international groups of experts to characterize the severity of acute renal failure by the following parameters (27.29):

- Mortality.
- Evolution towards extra-renal purification.
- Progression to chronic renal failure.
- Length of stay in intensive care.

Table 2: KDIGO criteria for assessing the severity of acute renal failure.

Stadium	Plasma creatinine	Diuresis
1	≥ 26.5 µmol/l or 1.5 to 1.9 times baseline plasma creatinine	< 0.5 ml/kg/h for 6 a.m. to 12 p.m.
2	2.0 to 2.9 times baseline plasma creatinine	< 0.5 ml/kg/h for ≥ 12h
3	3.0 times baseline plasma creatinine or plasma creatinine ≥ 354 pmol/l or initiation of renal replacement therapy	< 0.3ml/kg/h for ≥ 24h or anuria for ≥ 12h

(5)

The AKIN (Acute Kidney Injury Network) score (Table 3) uses diuresis as a clinical parameter and creatinineemia as a biological one (26):

Table 3: The AKIN score.

Stadium	***Creatininemia***	***Diuresis***
1	*Creates 1.5 to 2 x normal or increases by 26.4 µmole in 48h*	*<0.5ml/kg for 06heures*
2	*Creation x 2 to 3*	*<0.5ml/kg for 06heures*
3	*Créat > x3 or Créat >350 µmole or EER*	*<0.3ml/kg for 24h or Anuria >12 hours*

(26)

The KDIGO recommendations do not take muscle mass into account, which poses a problem for assessment in children (5). The modified RIFLE p RIFLE classification is much better suited to the paediatric population (Table 4).

Table 4: Modified RIFLE classification (paediatric).

Stadium	*Estimated plasma creatinine clearance*	*Diuresis*
Risk	*Decreased by >25*	*<0.5ml/kg/h for >8 h*
Injury	*Decreased by >50*	*<0.5ml/kg/h for >16 h*
Failure	*Decreased by >75% or <35/ml/min/1.73m²*	*<0.3ml/kg/h for 24 h or anuria for >12 h*
Loss (loss of function)	*Prolonged "Failure" stage > 4 weeks*	
End Stage (Chronic renal failure)	*Prolonged "Failure" stage > 3 months*	

(5)

7. PREVENTION OF ACUTE RENAL FAILURE IN INTENSIVE CARE UNITS

Preventing acute renal failure in the ICU and intensive care unit essentially involves identifying subjects at risk, managing general hemodynamics, and avoiding potentially nephrotoxic products.

7.1 Identifying subjects at risk :

The risk factors for the onset of acute renal failure are well known, and require careful screening (Table 5). Of all the risk factors, pre-existing renal damage appears to be the most reliable predictor of acute renal failure (30). A 10 ml/min reduction in creatinine clearance is associated with a significant increase in mortality (31).

Table 5: Identification of risk factors for acute renal failure.

Main risk factors for acute renal failure	
Terrain and pathologies	***Context***
Age >65	*Sepsis*
Chronic renal failure	*Hemodynamic instability*
Male sex	*The perioperative period*
The black race	*Emergency surgery*
BMI>40 KG/m	*Extensive burns*
Hypertension	*Polytrauma*
Congestive heart failure	*Use of nephrotoxic agents*
Hepatocellular insufficiency	
Severe respiratory insufficiency	
Diabetes	
Neoplastic pathologies	
Anemia	

(32)

7.2 Management of hemodynamics and optimization of oxygenation :

Renal blood flow and glomerular filtration rate are kept constant by effective mean arterial pressure (MAP). The Surviving Sepsis Campaign (4) recommends a MAP of 65 mmhg. These figures may vary according to age, the presence or absence of a history of arterial hypertension, and the local autoregulatory capacity of renal blood flow. The aim of mean arterial pressure (MAP) is to achieve a balance between vascular content and vascular volume (vascular resistance and blood volume). Blood volume is assessed by means of monitoring adapted to the resources and habits of each facility. However, the use of high-molecular-weight hydroxyethyl starch (Elohes, Voluven) leads to tubular osmotic nephrosis lesions and nephrotoxicity (33). Balanced solutions should probably be preferred in cases of heavy vascular filling, but without overloading, which is an independent factor in mortality. Vasopressors are commonly used to correct hemodynamic instability. However, it appears that the use of noradrenaline is much safer and less aggressive than the use of other alpha-effect amines (34, 35).

The terminal vascularization of the kidney and the cortico-medullary oxygen partial pressure gradient, with its highly uneven distribution of blood flow, explain the sensitivity of the renal parenchyma to ischemia (26). To combat this precarious balance in medullary oxygenation, several adaptive mechanisms have been described (Figure 5):

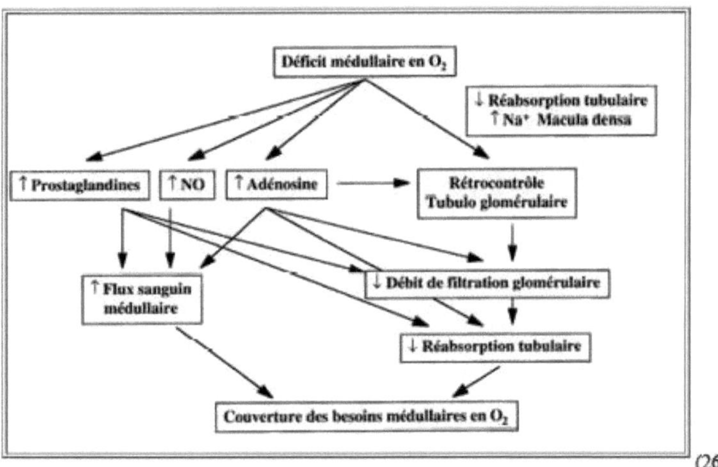

(26)

Figure 5: Regulation of renal medullary oxygenation.

The key to combating renal ischemia lies in managing general hemodynamics (mean arterial pressure) and local glomerular hemodynamics.

7.3 Avoidance of potentially nephrotoxic products:

Against a background of ongoing renal stress (inflammatory reactions, hemodynamic instability, organ failure), any additional stress, particularly toxic, can precipitate the onset of acute renal failure. Renal damage in the intensive care setting is mainly caused by drugs (36):

- Non-steroidal anti-inflammatory drugs (NSAIDs).
- Converting enzyme inhibitors and angiotensin II antagonists
- Aminoglycosides.
- Iodine for radiological examinations.

Additional examinations or the administration of potentially nephrotoxic drugs should not be delayed if they are essential to the patient's management. The use of crystalloid hydration to prevent nephropathy associated with iodinated contrast media can ideally be suggested before contrast injection and 6 hours afterwards. N-Acetylcysteine and/or sodium bicarbonate should not be used to prevent contrast-associated nephropathy.

Mechanical ventilation may contribute to kidney damage through the probable combination of several mechanisms (37)

- Reduced cardiac output due to altered myocardial loading conditions.
- Activation of the inflammatory system.
- Activation of the renin angiotensin aldosterone system.

In cases where aminoglycosides are indispensable, the rules for their use must be respected: administration in one injection per day, monitoring of residual levels beyond one injection, administration for a maximum of 3 days whenever possible.
NSAIDs, ARB2s and ACE inhibitors should be avoided in patients at risk of ARF.

8. PERIOPERATIVE ACUTE RENAL FAILURE

There is no consensus in the literature on the definition of perioperative acute renal failure. The KDIGO diagnostic criteria, based on creatinine levels and diuresis, can be used to define perioperative renal failure (38).

The perioperative period is particularly prone to kidney damage. AKI is often the result of several of these interrelated stresses. A distinction can be made between ARF of hemodynamic origin, ARF mediated by the inflammatory system, ARF of toxic cause and ARF of obstructive or "post-renal" origin.

Pre-renal damage is often the consequence of hypovolemia or renal congestion. Hypovolemia may be "true" or relative, in connection with vasoplegia induced by anesthetic drugs, or when a restrictive filling strategy is adopted, or when intraoperative losses are significant (bleeding, open surgery, duration of the operation).

Renal congestion linked to increased right-sided filling pressures, which influence perfusion of peripheral organs (CVP: central venous pressure).

Inflammation-mediated perioperative ARF shares certain pathophysiological features with ARF associated with sepsis. During surgery. This inflammatory cascade is aseptic in origin, but some of the mediators expressed have nephrotoxic properties. This mechanism is particularly well described during cardiothoracic surgery under extracorporeal circulation. The exclusively local inflammatory reaction of the renal parenchyma plays a major role in the development of AKI. Its pathophysiological mechanisms are complex and as yet incompletely understood.

Post-renal involvement should be suspected in patients undergoing urological or pelvic surgery (compression, obstruction, ureteral ligation). Organic parenchymal damage due to tubular necrosis may be suggested by prolonged hypoperfusion, hemolysis or the use of nephrotoxic drugs or products.

The prognosis of peri-operative renal damage is not entirely clear. It depends on the criteria used to define AKI and the visceral failures associated with renal failure.

9. NEPHRO PROTECTION

The use of a nephroprotection protocol significantly reduces the incidence of postoperative AKI (39). Some of the measures proposed in nephroprotection protocols, such as hemodynamic assessment or consultation with a nephrologist, are particularly time-consuming, and it is difficult to envisage their systematic application to all patients, irrespective of their individual risk of AKI. Nephroprotection protocols could be preferentially aimed at a population with an excess risk of progression to AKI (Table 6):

Table 6: Nephroprotection principles

	KDIGO 2012 measurements	RFE 2015
HEMODYNAMICS	*-Guarantee volume status and perfusion pressure: - shock, use isotonic crystalloids (2B) - Use vasopressors in conjunction with filling (1C) - Institute hemodynamic monitoring and a management protocol (2C) -Diuretics are not recommended to prevent AKI (1B)*	*Vascular filling : - Do not use hydroxyethyl starch (1-, strong) - Prefer crystalloids (2+, strong) - Prefer balanced solutions (2+, strong) Maintaining PAM : - Minimum level: 60 and 70 mmHg (1+, strong) - MAP > 70 mmHg for hypertensives (2+ strong) - Noradrenaline as first-line therapy to maintain MAP targets (2+, strong) Cardiac output : - Monitor and optimize systolic ejection volume or its derivatives (1+, strong) Avoid hydrosodium overload (2+, strong) Reserve diuretics for the treatment of the hydrosodium overload (1-, strong)*

NEPHROTOXICS MANAGEMENT	***Nephrotoxic products*** *:* *- Stop as soon as possible* ***Iodinated contrast media :*** *- Consider alternatives (NG)* *- Use low doses (NG)* *- Prefer iso- or hypoosmolar (1B)* *- Vascular filling with NaCl 0.9% or bicarbonates of sodium (1A)* *- Oral N-acetylcysteine and vascular filling (2C)* ***Aminosides :*** *- Avoid use unless there are no alternatives (2A) - 1 injection per day (2B), monitoring (1A)*	***Nephrotoxic :*** *Do not delay examinations or the administration of drugs if they are necessary for the patient's care (strong AE)* *Do not use NSAIDs, ACE inhibitors, ARB 2 (AE, strong)* ***Iodinated contrast media :*** *- Hydration (crystalloids) before injection, continued for 6 to 12 hours.* *12 hours (2+, strong)* *- Do not use N-acetylcysteine and/or sodium bicarbonate (2- strong)* ***Aminosides*** *(2+, strong):* *- 1 injection per day*
OTHER	*Target blood glucose: 6.1-8.3 mmol/l (2C)*	
PHARMACOLOGICAL TREATMENT	*Not recommended:* *Fenoldopam (2C), natriuretic factor (2C), recombinant human IGF-1 (1B), N-acetylcysteine (2D), dopamine (1A)*	*Not recommended:* *Sodium bicarbonate (2-, strong); mannitol, dopamine, fenoldopam, atrial natriuretic factor, N-acetylcysteine, insulin like growth factor-1, erythropoietin, adenosine receptor antagonists (1-, strong)*
MONITORING	*Monitor creatinine and diuresis*	*Monitor creatinine and diuresis*

10.THERAPEUTICS

In the presence of acute renal failure, the main question facing the practitioner in charge of the patient is whether or not extra-renal replacement therapy (ERT) is necessary. To date, no specific treatment has clearly reversed the course of acute renal failure, despite therapeutic advances in hemodynamic and stress management (40).

Extra-renal replacement therapy (ERT) is the only truly suppletive therapy available. The prescription of ERT in the ICU remains poorly defined, with it being initiated in 5 to 10% of ICU patients, and the ideal time for its initiation not clearly established.

There is a strong consensus on the need to initiate renal replacement therapy in life-threatening situations (Tab.10) (31) :

- Hyperkalemia.
- Severe acidosis.
- Overload situations.

Table 7: Indications for initiation of renal replacement therapy.

Indications for renal replacement therapy
Sodium water inflation: Oligo anuria < 200ml/12h Pulmonary edema resistant to medical treatment
Hydroelectrolytic and acid-base disorders: Hyperkalemia > 6.5 (refractory to medical treatment) Dysnatremia (<115 or > 160 meq/l) Severe metabolic acidosis Ph < 7.0)
Azotemia > 30 mmol/l with signs of poor tolerance
Some poisoning

(31)

According to current literature, there is no ideal time to stop extra-renal purification, nor is it possible to recommend a precise time to stop it (40).

The use of diuretics in acute renal failure, with the aim of transforming the evolution of anuric or oligo-anuric acute renal failure into diuresis-preserving ARF, is not recommended in view of the data in the medical literature. There is an absence of beneficial effects, and sometimes even a deleterious effect on the survival of intensive care patients (41, 42).

The only indication for the use of diuretics in this context is the association of fluid overload with acute renal failure.

In addition to etiological treatment, extra-renal purification can also be combined with hemodynamic optimization and the avoidance of potentially nephrotoxic products to prevent worsening renal damage.

The following treatments should not be used to prevent or treat ARF:

- Mannitol,
- Renal dopamine
- N-acetylcysteine,
- Bicarbonated serum

In the specific case of prevention of rhabdomyolysis-induced ARF, while the need for extensive vascular filling seems established (43-4)], the choice of solute type remains debated. There are theoretical benefits to the use of sodium bicarbonate (inhibition of intra-renal vasoconstriction, inhibition of lipid peroxidation and reduced myoglobin crystallization). This theoretical benefit does not allow us to assert the superiority of sodium bicarbonate over other filling solutions.

Undernutrition in patients with AKI is generally associated with a high incidence of infectious complications, prolonged hospitalization and mortality (45). Nutritional support for these assaulted patients with AKI should be similar to that of patients without AKI, to achieve the same energy goals, preserve muscle mass and reduce mortality (46).

An increase in plasma creatinine of more than 25% of the baseline value, six months after renal injury, and the absence of EER dependency in a patient after AKI, is a criterion for non-recovery of renal function. These patients should be considered at risk of developing chronic renal failure. The incidence of chronic renal failure after an acute attack is equal to 25.8/100 patient-years, and that of chronic end-stage renal failure to 6.6/100 patient-years. Clearly, there is a link between acute kidney injury and the risk of progression to chronic renal failure.

Patients with chronic renal failure are at particular risk of developing AKI on CKD, due to their lack of functional renal reserve. Measures to prevent AKI remain the same as for patients without CKD, and are based mainly on active and reinforced prevention, taking into account the elements mentioned above. Particular attention should be paid to monitoring nephrotoxic or renally eliminated treatments.

11. CONCLUSION

Peri-operative ARF is a frequent complication, particularly in cardiovascular surgery and in surgery involving significant volume loss. Its occurrence is associated with an increase in morbidity and mortality, and in the cost of the stay. In the absence of specific therapies for AKI, prevention and nephroprotection strategies must be implemented in patients at risk. Renal dysfunction should be monitored using two clinico-biological criteria: creatinine level and diuresis rate.

Preventive measures include identifying subjects at risk, managing the patient's general hemodynamics, and avoiding non-essential nephrotoxic products.

12.BIBLIOGRAPHY

1. Metnitz PG, Krenn CG, Steltzer H, Lang T, Ploder J, Lenz K, et al. Effect of acute renal failure requiring renal replacement therapy on outcome in critically ill patients. Critical care medicine. 2002;30(9):2051-8.

2. Nin N, Lombardi R, Frutos-Vivar F, Esteban A, Lorente JA, Ferguson ND, et al. Early and small changes in serum creatinine concentrations are associated with mortality in mechanically ventilated patients. Shock. 2010;34(2):109-16.

3. Mehta RL, Mcdonald B, Gabbai FB, Pahl M, Pascual MT, Farkas A, et al. A randomized clinical trial of continuous versus intermittent dialysis for acute renal failure. Kidney international. 2001;60(3):1154-63.

4. Uchino S, Kellum JA, Bellomo R, Doig GS, Morimatsu H, Morgera S, et al. Acute renal failure in critically ill patients: a multinational, multicenter study. Jama. 2005;294(7):813-8.

5. Ichai C, Vinsonneau C, Souweine B, Canet E, Clec'h C, Constantin J-M, et al. Acute renal failure in perioperative and intensive care (excluding extrarenal purification techniques). Intensive care medicine. 2017 ;26(6):481- 504.

6. Dieusaert P, Deweerdt L. Guide pratique des analyses médicales. Lyon Pharmaceutique. 1996;5(47):271.

7. Du Cheyron D, Terzi N, Charbonneau P. New biological markers of acute renal failure. Réanimation. 2008;17(8):775-82.

8. Lerolle N. Use of the renal vascular resistance index measured by Doppler ultrasound during septic shock. Réanimation. 2009;18(8):708-13.

9. Schnell D, Darmon M. What is the place of renal Doppler in the management of acute renal failure? Intensive Care Medicine. 2016;25(6):570-7.

10. Radermacher J, Mengel M, Ellis S, Stuht S, Hiss M, Schwarz A, et al. The renal arterial resistance index and renal allograft survival. New England Journal of Medicine. 2003;349(2):115-24.

11. Mostbeck GH, Zontsich T, Turetschek K. Ultrasound of the kidney: obstruction and medical diseases. European radiology. 2001;11(10):1878-89.

12. Audren N. Are renal vascular resistance index and Neutrophil Gelatinase Associated

Lipocalin assay markers of acute renal failure after cardiac surgery? 2012.

13. Darmon M, Schortgen F, Vargas F, Liazydi A, Schlemmer B, Brun-Buisson C, et al. Diagnostic accuracy of Doppler renal resistive index for reversibility of acute kidney injury in critically ill patients. Intensive care medicine. 2011;37(1):68-76.
14. Cooper CJ, Murphy TP, Cutlip DE, Jamerson K, Henrich W, Reid DM, et al. Stenting and medical therapy for atherosclerotic renal-artery stenosis. New England Journal of Medicine. 2014;370(1):13-22.
15. Granata A, Zanoli L, Clementi S, Fatuzzo P, Di Nicolò P, Fiorini F. Resistive intrarenal index: myth or reality? The British journal of radiology. 2014;87(1038):20140004.
16. Platt JF, Ellis JH, Rubin JM, DiPietro MA, Sedman AB. Intrarenal arterial Doppler sonography in patients with nonobstructive renal disease: correlation of resistive index with biopsy findings. AJR American journal of roentgenology. 1990;154(6):1223-7.
17. Platt JF, Rubin JM, Ellis JH. Acute renal failure: possible role of duplex Doppler US in distinction between acute prerenal failure and acute tubular necrosis. Radiology. 1991;179(2):419-23.
18. Sugiura T, Wada A. Resistive index predicts renal prognosis in chronic kidney disease. Nephrology Dialysis Transplantation. 2009;24(9):2780-5.
19. Parolini C, Noce A, Staffolani E, Giarrizzo GF, Costanzi S, Splendiani G. Renal resistive index and long-term outcome in chronic nephropathies. Radiology. 2009;252(3):888-96.
20. Onur MR, Cubuk M, Andic C, Kartal M, Arslan G. Role of resistive index in renal colic. Urological research. 2007;35(6):307-12.
21. Youssef DM, Fawzy FM. Value of renal resistive index as an early marker of diabetic nephropathy in children with type-1 diabetes mellitus. Saudi journal of kidney diseases and transplantation. 2012;23(5):985.
22. Ishimura E, Nishizawa Y, Kawagishi T, Okuno Y, Kogawa K, Fukumoto S, et al. Intrarenal hemodynamic abnormalities in diabetic nephropathy measured by duplex Doppler sonography. Kidney international. 1997;51(6):1920-7.
23. Masulli M, Mancini M, Liuzzi R, Daniele S, Mainenti P, Vergara E, et al. Measurement of the intrarenal arterial resistance index for the identification and

prediction of diabetic nephropathy. Nutrition, Metabolism and Cardiovascular Diseases. 2009;19(5):358-64.

24. Çelebi H, Donder E, Çeliker H. Renal blood flow detection with Doppler ultrasonography in patients with hepatic cirrhosis. Archives of internal medicine. 1997;157(5):564-6.
25. Joly D. Nephrology. In: Vernazobres-Grego, editor. ECN nephrology. 370. 2013 ed. Paris2013. p. 252.
26. P Jambou SK, D Grimaud. Perioperative renal protection. Conférences d'actualisation SFAR. 1996:p. 209-28.
27. . J-P Haymann, C Vinsonneau , A Girshovich. Acute obstructive renal failure: a pathophysiological reading. https://doi.org/10.1016/j.nephro.2017.01.008
28. Joannidis M, Metnitz B, Bauer P, Schusterschitz N, Moreno R, Druml W, et al. Acute kidney injury in critically ill patients classified by AKIN versus RIFLE using the SAPS 3 database. Intensive care
29. Coca SG, Singanamala S, Parikh CR. Chronic kidney disease after acute kidney injury: a systematic review and meta-analysis. Kidney international. 2012;81(5):442-8.
30. Lameire N, editor Which are the therapeutic interventions allowing to ensure a protection of the renal function? Annales francaises d'anesthesie et de reanimation; 2005.
31. Klouche K, Sandapa D, Barrau H, Jonquet O. Acute renal failure in intensive care-Prevention and treatment. Réanimation. 2011;20:552-9.
32. Kheterpal S, Tremper KK, Heung M, et al. Development and validation of an acute kidney injury risk index for patients undergoing general surgery: results from a national data set. Anesthesiology 2009;110:505-15
33. Schortgen F, Lacherade J-C, Bruneel F, Cattaneo I, Hemery F, Lemaire F, et al. Effects of hydroxyethylstarch and gelatin on renal function in severe sepsis: a multicentre randomised study. The lancet. 2001;357(9260):911-6.
34. Martin C, Papazian L, Perrin G, Saux P, Gouin F. Norepinephrine or dopamine for the treatment of hyperdynamic septic shock? Chest. 1993;103(6):1826-31.
35. Martin C, Viviand X, Leone M, Thirion X. Effect of norepinephrine on the outcome of septic shock. Critical care medicine. 2000;28(8):2758-65.

36. Dennen P1 DI, Anderson R. Acute kidney injury in the intensive care unit: an update and primer for the intensivist. Crit Care Med 2010;38 (1):261-75.
37. Pannu N, Mehta RL. Mechanical ventilation and renal function: an area for concern? American journal of kidney diseases. 2002;39(3):616-24.
38. Benchekroune S, Karpati PC, Berton C, et al. Diastolic arterial blood pressure: a reliable early predictor of survival in human septic shock. J Trauma 2008; 64:1188-95
39. Céline MONARD , Thomas RIMMELE. Preventing perioperative acute renal failure. https://doi.org/10.1016/j.anrea.2021.02.003
40. Thomas Rimmelé MD P. Acute Kidney Injury. SFAR. 2013.
41. Mehta RL, Pascual MT, Soroko S, Chertow GM, Group PS. Diuretics, mortality, and nonrecovery of renal function in acute renal failure. Jama. 2002;288(20):2547-53.
42. Uchino S, Doig GS, Bellomo R, Morimatsu H, Morgera S, Schetz M, et al. Diuretics and mortality in acute renal failure. Critical care medicine. 2004;32(8):1669-77.
43. Bosch X, Poch E, Grau JM. Rhabdomyolysis and acute kidney injury. N Engl J Med 2009;361:62-72
44. Scharman EJ, Troutman WG. Prevention of kidney injury following rhabdomyolysis: a systematic review. Ann Pharmacother 2013;47:90-105
45. Uchino S, Kellum JA, Bellomo R, et al. Acute renal failure in critically ill patients: a multinational, multicenter study. JAMA 2005;294:813-818
46. Cano N, Aparicio M, Brunori G, Carrero JJ, Cianciaruso B, Fiaccadori E et al. ESPEN Guidelines on Parenteral Nutrition: adult renal failure. Clin Nutr 2009;28:401-14

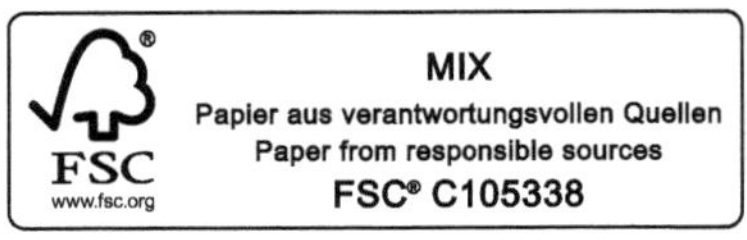

Printed by Books on Demand GmbH, Norderstedt / Germany